I Love Coconut Oil:
56 Simple Tips
for Everyday Use

Cricket Desmarais

sea star press . key west . florida

Published by

sea star press
p.o. box 4038
key west, fl 33040
www.ilovecoconutoil.com

copyright 2011 by Cricket Desmarais

Desmarais, Cricket
I Love Coconut Oil: 56 Simple Tips For Everyday Use
ISBN-13: 978-0615508412 (Custom)
ISBN-10: 0615508413
BISAC: Health & Fitness / Healthy Living

Dedicated to my family —
& to you & yours.

Table of contents

Part two: Let the uses begin!

I said "Doctor, ain't there nothing I can take?"

I said "Doctor, to relieve this bellyache?

Harry Nilsson, "Coconut"

Foreword

The low-fat diet revolution of the 80s took hold from the overly simplistic governmental and medical advice that dietary fat makes us fat and is the cause of stroke and cardiovascular disease. The guidelines did not distinguish between good fats and bad and simply told us that "fat is bad."

We followed doctor's advice and switched from butter to "heart healthy" margarine and from saturated lard fats to unsaturated and polyunsaturated corn oil and soy oil fats. We threw out our egg yolks for fear of cholesterol and began consuming truckloads of sugar-laced, low-fat and no-fat foods.

The result has been a skyrocketing epidemic of obesity, stroke and heart disease, along with hormonal imbalances, immune problems and a whole host of good fat deficiency syndromes and bad fat metabolic dysfunctions.

Thankfully, more and more people are finally re-awakening to the fact that there are good fats and bad fats. People know that good fats, like omega-3 fatty acids, found in flax seed and fish oils, are important to health and that bad fats, like the highly processed unnatural "trans fats", harm us by damaging the membranes of the very cells that we are made of.

Unfortunately, many of us remain unaware of, or still think badly of, pure coconut oil.

Cricket Desmarais is helping to correct this problem and has given us a wonderful gift in I Love Coconut Oil: 56 Simple Tips for Everyday Use, in which she clearly and simply explains the many, many "near miracle" health benefits that can be had from pure, raw, humble coconut oil.

"Coconut oil is not only one of the good fats - it is the best of the best"

Ross Williams, DC
Doctor of Chiropractic, Clinical Nutritionist

From the author

Before I begin, please allow me to "confess" that I am not a celebrity, an expert, or any sort of official authority on nutrition, health or wellness.

I say "confess" in jest, because I believe that practical advice on how to simply and safely incorporate coconut oil in a day-to-day way could actually come from someone who is doing her best to take good care of her family and herself by educating herself and making as many good choices as possible — with no alliances towards any product or potential research funding.

Someone who has tried coconut oil in every way shape and form possible for themselves in the last five years to discover the many benefits *first hand*. That's where I come in.

It started with a quest for good health, a clear mind, and a radiant inner and outer beauty. We all want that, don't we?

And yet, most of us live in a world where there are boundless avenues that veer us away from such things, or worse, bombard us with health opinions or options wrapped in glossy packages— touting false claims that we dutifully believe because we so desperately want to feel and look better.

Here's the good news: it doesn't have to be so difficult. In fact, nature offers us something so simple as a way of helping us get there, and it's found in none other than— the coconut.

Yes, the implicit, simple health found within the coconut makes paving the way to healing and happiness all that much easier and more hopeful.

Right now you might be thinking "*What?! Health and hope from a coconut?!*"

While it may sound a bit grand, it's true. I'd even go so far as to say coconut oil changed my life. Not coconut oil alone, per se, but what I experienced and learned as I used it.

Amid the maze of nutritional information that has bombarded me along my path to healing, coconut oil has been a key ingredient along that journey. The more I learn about it, the more I learn about the balance of my own body and how certain choices support or negate my overall health and wellness. As they say, knowledge is power, especially when acted upon.

I'll admit, there was a time when I

wasn't exactly a fan of the fuzzy nut or what came out of it. Sure, I'd delight in a macaroon drenched in chocolate, drift off into vacation reverie with the slightest whiff of coconut-scented tanning oil and occasionally indulge in a pina colada when traveling the tropics. But that's about as far as my coconut-inducing days went.

In fact, I was completely unaware of any health or wellness the coconut or its oil offered. I was a product of my childhood environment, which did not include coconuts but a swirling myriad of quick fixes, passing fads, the hype of fast foods and microwave meals and a mélange of antibiotics.

And to top it off, in the past two-plus decades, I was always on the go and eager to succeed, stopping at nothing to get there. Stress coursed through my veins as did the mantras "prove yourself" and "work harder."

That is, until my health began to rapidly decline and my body began to resist or reject any strain of antibiotic prescribed to assist me.

Doctors were unable to pinpoint my problem, and my kidneys and bladder were exploding with toxicity. I could scarcely walk in public without fear that I might wet myself because of the constant barrage of urinary tract infections I was having.

In total surrender, I visited a local health food store, pleading with the staff to point me in the right direction. On one of the shelves I found a book about body ecology and entered the phase of my life that I'll now term "food and chemical recovery." It was a powerful journey into knowing that I had the opportunity to make choices that would either support- or stifle- my wellness.

With proper nutrition and food balancing coupled with other alternative modalities, I began to reclaim my health and discovered how to best deal with what I realized was Candida and overall poor nutrition.

Still, I hadn't discovered coconut oil until one practically hit me on the head in Key West.

It was a friendly metaphoric toss from a friend who sold his eco-friendly and indigenous landscaping company to pursue a degree in natural nutrition and the making of fair-trade extra virgin coconut oil. I'd always admired his entrepreneurial spirit and knowledge of nutrition, so of course I was intrigued about his fixation on coconuts and their oil.

He gave me a starter kit—a gallon of his Cocopura product and told me to have at it, and like the health store crew from a decade previous, pointed me to certain books where I might learn of some of the healthful benefits of this oil.

While reading those books have been quite helpful and have led me deeper down the rabbit hole of cyber research on all things coconut oil, the real benefits have come from experiencing it first hand.

Every day for the last five years, I have reached for coconut oil in either my kitchen or my bathroom. And since then, I've seen it boost my immunity, heal wounds, decrease the adversity of a bout with illness or prevent an illness altogether.

I've tossed out the majority of my beauty products, slathering the oil on my face and body and applying it moderately to my hair while also ingesting two to three tablespoons daily.

My once acne-prone and sun-damaged skin is now smooth and soft, with flare-ups only occurring when I'm out of balance or, ahem… in my cycle. My former brittle hair is now thick, shiny and strong, and the pain in my joints from Candida inflammation is near gone. I would even go so far as to say that I believe my daily intake of coconut oil more than likely increased my fertility and previous problems with endometriosis, and now, with two toddlers in tote, our family is most often healthy and well, all of us benefiting from the many uses of coconut oil.

This isn't to say I haven't had to make some serious changes in my overall attitude and lifestyle and that everything happened because of coconut oil alone. That would be a terrible untruth and disservice to you.

The fact is I've had to look long and hard at all of my lifestyle choices and continuously check in with my self to see if what I was saying "yes" to was actually saying "yes" back to me.

Sure, I love a Cuban con leche (with sugar) from our famous little laundro-mat down the street, but is it adding to my health and wellness?

Are those sides of French fries with my good-for-me veggie burger really the complement to my "healthy" lunch?

Does saying yes to staying up too late

to get more work done really amount to a greater increase by week's end, when I am feeling run-down and haggard?

Though I believe in the divine perfection within, as the old saying goes—"nobody's perfect." Ultimately we all decide what's best for us in any given moment, and live (or suffer!) the consequences.

As much as I admire the purists out there and consider myself a highly conscious being, I am very much a part of this modern culture, enjoying the amenities and high-speed technology just as much as most people. Slowing down and taking stock of what is simple is the first step towards cultivating a higher awareness towards oneself and one's choices.

Coconut oil is one of the very things that helped me do just that.   I share this with you because it is my deep belief that you should reap the benefits of coconut oil and heightened health awareness, too.

There is so much information out there to help guide us to the road to wellness— it can all be a bit daunting.

The thing I love about coconut oil (among many things) is that it is an all-natural food, with no adverse side affects.

Even better is that when you take it for one particular reason, it will inevitably affect the greater whole, all in a positive and supportive manner. If you add coconut oil to any well-balanced, mindful health regime, you'll be sure to experience some shifts from within.

To best make sense of all the information I've gleaned from personal research, I've tried my best to put the many uses of coconut oil into appropriate sections with easy-to-read instructions.

All of the uses listed are simple and straight-forward, and can quickly be introduced to your lifestyle with relative ease and comfort.

You may find some resonate more than others, or some do not resonate at all. Experiment for yourself and see. Part of the journey towards wellness is learning how to distinguish what your body responds to and what it doesn't.

If you do have major health issues, of course you'd want to speak with your health care provider on any major or daily changes. He or she might even tell you about all the new research going on that shows just how healing coconut oil IS for many different types of chronic and debilitating diseases.

Should you be further interested in the many facets of coconut oil and want to get into the informative and scientific, nitty-gritty details, there are several references listed at the back of this book, including the fantastic offerings of Dr. Bruce Fife's website: www.coconutresearchcenter.org.

With a little information, guidance, encouragement and mindfulness, we all have the power to heal ourselves.

May hope, health and happiness be yours!

Introduction

If you were offered a simple, low-cost, non-toxic, all-natural method towards wellness, would you take it? What if it were a prescription-free, over-the-counter remedy with dozens of practical applications that would optimize your health?

No such thing, you say? Well, consider the coconut— or more specifically, the oil that comes from it.

Yes, coconut oil!

An age-old tropical topical and ingestible antidote for more than just a few ailments, this curative oil has innumerable benefits. Immune boosting, skin protecting, digestion improving, anti-aging, weight loss stimulating and disease preventing are just a few of the therapeutic properties of what some nutritionists call "the perfect food." Ingesting three to four tablespoons a day could change your health dramatically, especially if supported by better lifestyle choices all-around.

The benefits of coconut oil have been scientifically studied as far back as the fifties. That's more than a half a century worth of medical research, published studies and clinical observations that support the miracles of this so-called miracle oil.

In fact, it shares some of the same fatty acids found in breast milk, which modern doctors recommend newborns be fed for at least the first year of their life. Converted by the body, these life-propelling **lauric acid** liquids (which we'll discuss in a later chapter) provide protection against viral, bacterial and protozoal infections. And—in both breast milk and coconut oil— that's just the start of things. The clinical list of what these medium chain fatty acids found in coconut oil can do is virtually endless.

Even when one looks beyond our "prove it to me" society (just the facts and figures, thank you very much!), there are plenty of living testaments based among the peoples of Asia, the Pacific Islands, Africa and Central America that have been holding steady for thousands of years.

Think about it—how often do they suffer from our modern degenerative diseases? Heart disease? Diabetes? Cancer? While the rest of the western world is plagued by a bevy of diseases, pains and problems, these native people thrive in good health and good spirits.

Sadly, when they embrace the western ways and abandon their own instinctive eating habits, their health begins to deteriorate, mirroring diseases that reflect the diets westerners are so well-known for. "Super-size me" and "fat-free" products become paradoxical to the people living in tropical paradises.

It's literally the indigenous diets of these people that keep them vibrantly alive, with strong bodies and clear, glowing skin despite the harsh sun and other weather elements. And, not so coincidentally, the common food factor is—you guessed it—lots and lots of coconuts!

Unfortunately, the marketing efforts of

competitive industries have created myths and misrepresentations of coconut oil. Misnomers and political propaganda about the healthiest oil on earth were created by self-serving commercial enterprises (enter the American Soybean Association) that swept us up into skepticism. Their job was to help the soybean soar, and that they did with their media blitz against all other oils, including that of the coconut.

When all was said and done, people were left wondering how a saturated fat, the prime proponent for heart attacks, was good for them. The American Soybean Association helped brand coconut oil as one of the end-all-be-all culprits to bad health, a reflection not based on facts but on "money, politics, and misunder-standing," says nutritionist and naturopathic doctor Bruce Fife, world authority on coconut oil and coconuts.

Fife has penned several books about the myths and miracles of coconut oil, complete with details on understanding fats and the medicinal and cosmetic benefits that come from it. His books have been instrumental in helping me delve deeper into understanding the WHY in coconut's amazing healing properties and I recommend reading them if you feel called to do dig deeper yourself.

With the help of research from folks like Fife and other truth-seeking scientists, the healing secrets of coconut oil are finally coming to the forefront of modern medical science. Their discoveries are amazing and virtually endless, and the studies proliferate medical journals and the internet with a constant stream of positive results.

We do, however, recognize that every body is different, with its own set of genetics creating or challenging our health. This book isn't meant to be cavalier towards those that struggle with serious medical issues, nor is it to replace any medical counseling, medications or serve as a stand-alone treatment for any serious health conditions you may be suffering.

What is offered here is information, in an easy-to-use fashion, about coconut oil and all that it can do to support you towards health and wellness.

The bottom line is this: coconut oil — when mindfully applied within a balanced lifestyle — provides an inexpensive and harmless way to propagate wellness within our own bodies. Only you-- and your health care provider if you are working with one-- know what is best for you. We encourage you to explore the uses and decide if they resonate.

Whether experimented with and employed from your kitchen cupboard, your medicine cabinet, your beauty regime, or a variety of other surprising and simple ways, coconut oil is truly a unique and powerful ingredient that will boost the vibration in both your body and your home.

In the pages that follow, we offer you 56 straightforward ways to try it and see for yourself.   Feel free to jump ahead or skip what doesn't seem right. There's no rule or methodology to what ought to come first or last.

As with most things, if you make it fun, you will likely find your experiences more successful.   And remember, the daily aspect of consciously using coconut oil will make you more conscious overall, thereby making you more in tune with yourself and your choices. How fortunate we are to have so many. Here's to making the ones that serve our health best!

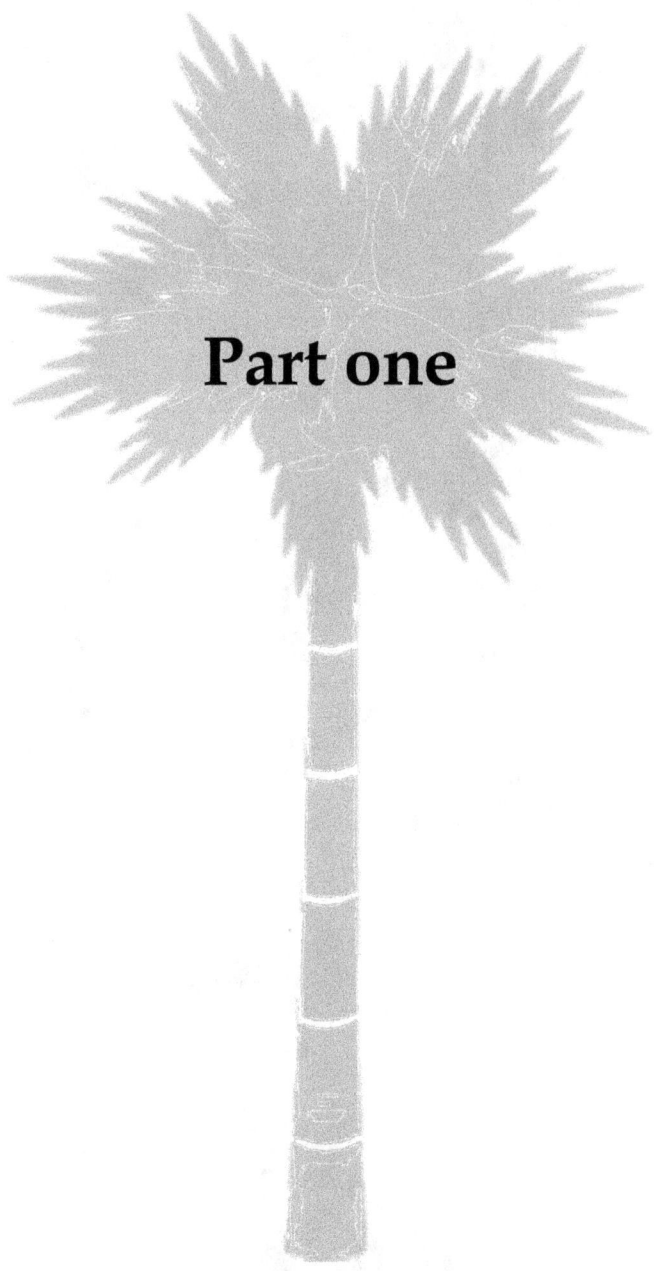

Part one

De-mystifying science: Cracking the nut on why *this* saturated fat is actually good for you

How can a saturated fat be GOOD for you? We've been told time and again that saturated fats are anything but, increasing obesity and cardiovascular disease and a slew of other health issues.

But wait—that was based on research from decades ago, right? Now, they're booing the same polyunsaturated fats (vegetable oils) once urged upon us to help us combat cholesterol? The conflicting information is enough to make your head spin! It's no wonder so many do their darndest to avoid fats altogether. Which is, in fact, another mistake.

Let's take a closer look at fats, especially those found in coconut oil. By better understanding how fats function in our bodies, we'll see how fats are actually essential to our systems, and how coconut oil can be an incredible benefit to our overall health, regulating all of the body's functions while also improving and building immunity.

Take a deep breath while we dive into the deep end of the science pool.

The major functions of fat are to provide energy and cell structure for the body, so eliminating them is not the wisest option.

All fats and oils are made up of fat molecules— or fatty acids— which are classified based on their saturation (saturated, polyunsaturated and monounsaturated) and the molecular length of the carbon chain within the fatty acid. Fatty acids help move oxygen through the bloodstream, are essential to cell membrane development, strength and function, and are vital to our organs and tissues.

Now, three fatty acids joined together have what are called triglycerides. Got all that? Good, because now we're going to do a very brief overview on the long, medium and short of them all.

Most fats from our diets come from long chain fatty acids, made up from things like lard, chicken fat and just about every vegetable oil out there.

But not coconut oil! Coconut oil is made up of MEDIUM chain fatty acids.

So, what's the difference, right? Do a few carbon chains really matter that much? The resounding answer is YES! It's all about absorption, digestion and metabolism, which are three key factors in helping the rest of our bodily functions function effectively.

Unlike long-chain triglycerides (LCT's), which require enzymes and bile for digestion and break down into lipoproteins (which break down via the bloodstream and body into artery-clogging fat cells!), medium-chain triglycerides (MCT's) do not need these enzymes for digestion and are immediately sent to and absorbed by the liver, where it quickly produces energy.

To put it more simply, long-chain

triglycerides have more work to do to break down into something useful, typically with an unwanted residue (i.e. slow-to-go, disease-causing fat), whereas medium-chain triglycerides deliver instant, clean energy for your body. Now that's efficiency!

That said, as with any type of fat, you want to be sure you don't overdo it. Fat is fat is fat when you aren't smart about it—we're not here to promote chugging down a cup of coconut oil every day and more isn't always better. Should you have pressing health issues, consult your physician about adding any supplemental health components to your diet.

Essential Fatty Acids: Three good reasons to use coconut oil

So now that you have a better understanding of the role of fats in coconut oil, let's dive a little deeper and see exactly what sort of fats we are dealing with.

We know they are medium-chain triglycerides, and that they bypass storage in the liver for immediate energy usage. Let's take a look at the active ingredients that contribute to that energy, found in the fatty acids. There are three in particular that pack the power into coconut oil.

The fatty acid content of coconut oil is: Caprylic (C8:0) 7.8 %, Capric (C10:0) 6.7%, and Lauric (C12:0) 47.5 %. Potent antimicrobial agents, these medium-chain fatty acids serve as warriors that disintegrate the cell walls of bacterial, viral and fungal invaders.

Let's look at them each individually to better understand the power of them combined.

Caprylic acid, or octanoic acid, is found in the milk of various mammals, in coconut and in palm oil. Its many uses are surprisingly rampant. Wherever you go in the public realm, capylic acid's presence is highly likely — and welcomed.

An antimicrobial pesticide used for sanitizing food contact surfaces, this amazing medium chain triglyceride is used with dairy equipment, food processing equipment, breweries, wineries, and beverage processing plants. Let's raise a toast to coconut oil.

That said, it shouldn't be surprising to see that it is also used as a disinfectant in organizations and institutions. Your local hospital is likely using it, as is the elementary school, your veterinarian, the restaurant you ate at last night and the hotel you will be staying at during your next vacation.

Those with a green thumb might already know about caprylic acid's abilities as an algaecide, bactericide and fungicide, as it is widely used in the nursery and landscape industry.

Medically speaking, caprylic acid has been used by many a physician to successfully treat Candida yeast infections, working especially well for those who have adverse reactions to anti-fungal drugs. So potent and powerful, it is even extracted and sold as a natural antifungal.

Because of its short chain length, it can easily penetrate a fatty cell wall membrane, making it effective in combating bacterial infections, like staphylococcus aureus and some species of streptoccus. See the correlation on how it helps keep things clean and supports life-enhancing growth?

Also occurring in coconut oil, palm kernel oil and the milk of some mammals is **capric acid**, also known as decanoic acid.

With strong antiviral and antimicrobial properties, it is converted into monocaprin in the body and helps combat viruses, bacteria and the yeast Candida Albicans. Coconut oil is one of the richest sources of capric acid, which has also been proven to assist in insulin regulation, inactivating parasites, aiding in gallbladder disease & the HIV virus. It, like caprylic acid, is also used as an antimicrobial pesticide in commercial food handling.

Let's get to the biggie of the three: **lauric acid,** which comprises more than half of what coconut oil is made up of. You may have even have heard of it, as it is most commonly used in the production of soaps and cosmetics.

Because it exhibits strong antimicrobial properties, it is also embraced by pharmaceutical companies that prepare antimicrobial drugs.

Then there is breastfeeding. The

medium chain fatty acids in breast milk and the nourishment they offer are considered so vital for a child's growth and development that even government-regulated institutions like the American Academy of Pediatrics encourage mothers to nurse their babies for at least the first year of life. (The World Health Organization emphasizes the importance of nursing up to two years of age and beyond). The primary fatty acid in breast milk? You guessed it— lauric acid— the same component in coconut oil that is now being studied for all of its own immune-boosting, antibacterial, antiviral, antifungal, and antiparasitic properties.

Nutritionist and biochemist Mary Enig,
one of the world's leading authorities on oils and fats, explains that lauric acid has the beneficial function of

being formed into monolaurin in the body.

She explains monolaurin as "the antiviral, antibacterial, and antiprotozoal monoglyceride used by the human or animal to destroy lipid coated viruses such as HIV, herpes, cytomegalovirus, influenza, various pathogenic bacteria including listeria monocytogenes and heliobacter pylori, and protozoa such as giardia lamblia."

That said, the correlation between lauric acid and its nutriceutical effects are—no pun intended—easy to digest. Combine all three of these medium chain fatty acids and what you get is a powerful proponent to your health. If that seems like too bold a statement, a little investigation into modern research will help set the tone of this truth quicker than you can say "I love coconut oil."

Allergy Alert: Is it a Nut or Not?

That's a really good question. It might seem obvious, being that the word "nut" is half of what makes up the word "coconut." But the fact of the matter is, categorizing the coconut has actually been quite controversial, and the answer not all that clear.

The Food and Drug Administration will tell you, as of 2006, that *yes*— coconut is a tree nut, and requires that any food made with them be listed visibly on the package.

A botanist will get nitty gritty with

you, detailing how it can technically be considered a fruit, a seed and a nut. More specifically, it is a fibrous one-seeded drupe, or a dry drupe, with a drupe defined as a fruit in which an outer fleshy part surrounds a shell.

Foods that are close biological relatives often share related allergenic proteins. Since coconuts are most closely related to other types of palms and betel and not to most other tree nuts, it is somewhat safe to say that people who are allergic to nuts won't necessarily be allergic to coconuts.

Somewhat. Because there are hazelnuts. And walnuts, too. There IS some evidence of cross-reactivity between coconuts and hazelnuts and coconuts and walnuts — in one patient during a June 2007 study as listed in the Annals of Allergy, Asthma and Immunology.

Clear as mud, right? If you have allergic tendencies, you just want to know if you can eat and use coconut oil, right?

With an estimated 1.8 million Americans experiencing allergies to tree nuts, haphazardly indulging in a sudden love for coconut oil might night be the best road to travel down if you are among that pack. Even if medical literature shows that the small amount of documented cases of coconut allergies are most often experienced by those who do NOT have former nut allergies.

And even if the studies show that adverse reactions are rare and not serious in those that DO experience them, the best thing you can do if you are highly prone to allergies with nuts and other foods is to check in with your allergist and go from there.

Getting started: Selecting your coconut oil

So you've read this far and have decided that you'd like to investigate the wellspring and wellness of coconut oil. Congratulations!

Now you're probably thinking, "Where do I begin?" Of course, that all depends on who you are and where you're hoping to head.

For one person, it may be simply to add a new flavor to their culinary repertoire. Another's needs may be more dire, hoping to help quell the ache of a difficult disease.

Whatever the case may be, this book was written to assist folks in figuring out how coconut oil can help them and just how simply it can be used. Every day.

While there are several companies that offer many great products, we recommend seeking out the extra virgin, cold-pressed variety. Raw, pure and organic, of course, is also recommended, as are those that come from ethical "fair trade" practices, ensuring that the people involved in its manufacturing and production are provided a fair wage and human working conditions.

Methods of production vary from one company to another and a little research will go a long way in helping you make your selection. While any type of virgin coconut oil will reap benefits, it is best to avoid oils that have been refined, bleached and deodorized (RBD). And you absolutely DO NOT want to use partially hydrogenated coconut oil. Any partially hydrogenated coconut oil creates trans fats, destroying the essential fatty acids, antioxidants and other positive elements of virgin coconut oil.

The three types of higher quality oils are traditional hand pressed/home made, DME (direct micro expeller), and premium virgin oils, all which have virtuous benefits, though premium oils offer the least amount of processing so that the natural vitamin E, antioxidants and fresh coconut "essence" are retained.

Whichever type of oil you go with, confirm that they aren't subjected to temperatures over 115F to be confident of the quality of production.

Because plastics can, at the molecular

level, leach out and mix with coconut oil, it is best when purchased in dark/amber glass jars that protect it from light and oxygen, helping it maintain its molecular integrity and all the benefits that come along with it.

Or look for high quality recyclable PET plastics (polyethylene terephthalate) for packaging, as they are non-leaching and will retain all that's good without negative alterations to the product within.

Of course, it helps to take note of where the coconuts come from when considering freshness.

For example, if you live in California, it may make better sense to get your coconut oil from a company who gets their coconuts from nearby Mexico, just as if you live in Australia, coconuts from New Zealand aren't too far of a hop, skip and a jump away from home, so they don't run the risk of spending several weeks in transport before they get to their production hub.

In short, the longer it takes for the coconuts to travel to their production destination, the chances of molding increase. Every bit of freshness counts.

When it comes to taste, if you try several varieties, you will notice that different products have different flavors- some bold, sweet, or delicate. If you plan on using your oil as a compliment to your cuisine, you might start with a more delicate flavor so as to enhance rather than hinder the other flavors you are bringing to the table.

Delicately flavored coconut oil is also a fine way to introduce yourself to its many uses, since it is easier on the palate and doesn't leave a strong aftertaste.

If you're still not sure which coconut oil is the one for you, experimenting with a variety in smaller jars might help you hone in on your favorite.

When you find one you really like, there are usually options to buy it in gallon-sized buckets, which will be cost effective and more convenient in the long run if you intend on using it daily, which of course, we highly recommend so as to get the optimal benefits.

And don't worry about it going "bad" on you...if you do choose to make coconut oil a part of your daily intake, it won't be long before it's gone. Since coconut oil is naturally saturated, it is highly resistant to rancidity and perioxidation. Most have a pretty long shelf life, meaning more than a year.

Whether you do a little internet research or visit your local health food store and see what's on the shelves, once you get the coconut oil into your home there are a few ways of making it more accessible for daily use.

If the oil keeps above 76-78 degrees at a standard room temperature, chances are likely that your oil will be in liquid form, so a funnel can come in handy when it comes to transferring the oil from the jar into easier-to-use receptacles.

Try a glass hand-soap pump for the bathroom and beauty uses, or an oil bottle with a spout for the kitchen. Oil spray bottles— both for the kitchen or for your aromatherapy needs— work great, too.

If you live in a cooler climate, you'll notice that your oil has a creamier, more solidified consistency, sometimes referred to as coconut "butter." Simply scoop it out in its solid form or put the container in a bowl of hot water to liquefy it as needed. If you plan on just plunging your fingers in for "beauty" needs, be sure to purchase a separate jar for kitchen duty to keep your food free from any contaminates.

While coconut oil does have a long shelf life, once it is opened it is best to use it within two months or refrigerate it if room temperature tends to be higher than 75 degrees. Chances are, however, that it'll take no time at all to go through your oil once you open it, as the myriad of uses will make it disappear quickly.

In either its liquid or solid form, on the inside of your body or on the out— coconut oil is considered one of the healthiest oil on earth, offering a broad spectrum of benefits from its naturally produced compounds.

Your coconut oil purchase is a promise to yourself that your journey towards health and wellness can be natural, flavorful, and fun.

A "miracle" cure, beauty aid & overall well-being balancer — everything can be backed up by published medical studies that now dot the world wide web and many medical journals. But the best proof is to use it yourself and be your own walking testimony.

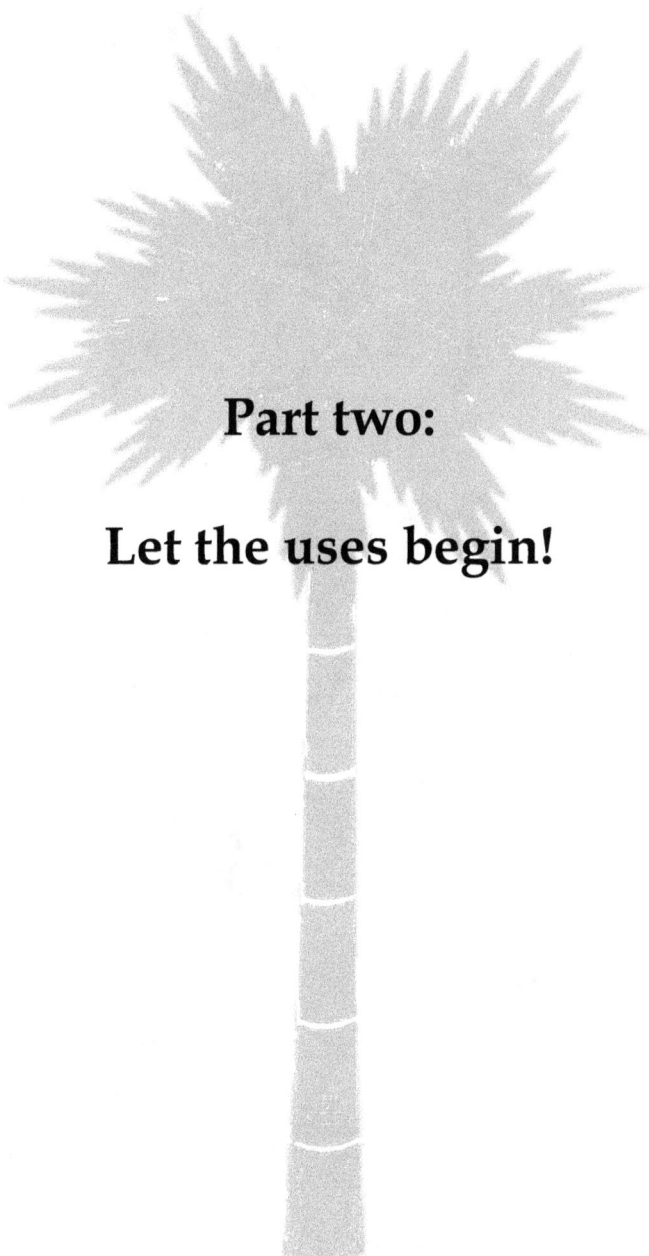

Part two:

Let the uses begin!

Good eats:
Creative culinary treats

Superfood to the rescue! A super what? A superfood— a natural food source highly concentrated with a complex supply of quality essential nutrients and rich in phytochemicals — that helps us reach optimum health and reduce the risk of disease.

With its rich natural source of medium-chain triglycerides (MCTs), coconut oil qualifies as a superfood, so eat it up.

Eating coconut oil is the number one way to receive all of its amazing benefits, so whether you add it to the well-balanced meals you are already eating or simply eat a few tablespoons of it each day, you will begin to feel the difference.

Did we mention that the medium chain triglycerides found in coconut oil also have antibacterial, antiviral, antifungal & anti-parasitic properties, which enhance the absorption of minerals and vitamins? Yet another reason to pour it on! All this and it tastes really good too!

1.

Sauté, fry, & stir-fry

If you do anything, shift this: your use of standard vegetable oils in the kitchen to your use of coconut oil. Not only will you help yourself shed any unwanted weight and easily boost your immunity, you will likely delight in the taste of your favorite foods prepared with coconut oil.

With a smoke point of 280 Fahrenheit, coconut oil has the highest flash point of all oils, meaning it will retain its natural structure and all of its nutritive benefits along with it when heated. That alone ought to be reason enough to consider trading out your old cooking oils for coconut oil.

Any veggie will taste great sautéed in coconut oil, and pancakes and grilled cheese sandwiches made with coconut oil (especially adored by my toddlers) are simply delicious.

Trust me, the switch will be well worth it in a myriad of ways, and you'll hardly even realize what a big switch you've made.

2.
Baker's delight

Try substituting whatever fat is recommended in your baked sweets recipe by 50% coconut oil (and any dairy with coconut milk) for a healthier, richer version.

Or lightly spray or drizzle on thinly sliced baked sweet potatoes for a yummy alternative to French fries. Get creative and you'll find the options are tastily endless.

3.
Boost your food

A tablespoon or two added to your soups, smoothies, or even oatmeal will help you along in your recommended daily intake (three and a half tablespoons for adults) as well as help your energy rise.

As previously mentioned, any vitamin powders used to make a smoothie will only be enhanced and better absorbed because of the addition of coconut oil.

4.

Dress your lettuce

No need for bottled salad dressings with ingredients you're not even sure you can pronounce. Simply toss your salads with a little bit of coconut oil and a combination of herbs, spices, lime or lemon that please your personal palate.

Coconut oil will harden when it touches cold vegetables, so if you prefer a more liquid version of your dressing, use half olive oil with half coconut oil to help stabilize the liquidity.

5.
Drizzle it

...on your popcorn, pastas, grains & potatoes. Move over butter, there's something better. If you're looking for something more health conscious and tasty to amp up the flavor, look no further. Coconut oil to the rescue.

Beauty & personal care: Nature's spa in a bottle

It's human nature to want to look & feel good — with coconut oil you can do both in a natural, non-toxic & eco-friendly way. When used as a tropical topical it softens the skin, protects it against damage, promotes healing and lends a vibrant, youthful glow.

Adding it to your diet is an even better option since the health of your skin is often the result of what's from within.

Either way, adding this oil with its three powerful antioxidants (vitamin E, phenol and phytosterol) will help reduce the number of free radicals in your skin and body, which will only translate into wellness on the inside and out.

This all-in-one oil is non-greasy, super absorbent & can be mixed with other essential oils for additional aroma-therapeutic benefits and sensational scents.

Lastly, consider this: your skin is not only your biggest organ, but it's extremely absorbent. If you can't eat it, why would you put it on your skin?

6.

All-over moisturizer

Every bit of your body will benefit from this oil that regenerates & nourishes the skin and promotes an all-over radiant glow.   Slather it on daily and watch dryness disappear. A little goes a long way, so experiment with amounts until you get what's right for your specific needs.

7.
Wrinkle diminisher

Loaded with antioxidants, coconut oil limits free radical damage to the skin when taken both internally and externally.

Replace the unsaturated fats in your diet with coconut oil while slathering it on your skin and experience the anti-aging benefits.

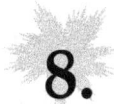

8.
Blemish blaster

While there are many causes for acne - ranging from hormones to stress to environment- often it is the result of systems on the inside going awry.

Internally ingesting coconut oil (3 1/2 tablespoons daily) helps maintain the balance of intestinal flora, which aids in digestion and reduction of acne-inducing yeast in the body.

The antimicrobial properties found in coconut oil also boost the concentration of lauric acid on our skin, which helps deter acne-causing bacteria.

Topically or internally, coconut oil is worth a try, and unlike antibiotics — which when used over a long period of time — won't compromise your immune system's natural ability to heal itself.

I like to add a little tea tree oil to troublesome spots when they do appear, penetrating more deeply while giving an aroma-therapeutic boost.

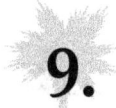

9.
Low maintenance manicure & pedicure

Save time and money with this simple approach to keeping your hands and feet smooth and sweet. Mix a half a cup of sugar with 2 tablespoons of coconut oil and a dash of peppermint oil in a bowl, then massage into your feet and hands. Rinse with warm water. Old skin will slough away, cuticles will soften, and your extremities will tingle with the attention you've given them. For deeper treatments, finish off with extra oil and a nightcap of cotton socks or gloves.

10.
Make-up remover

Why douse your dear face with a slew of ingredients you can scarcely pronounce? A dab of oil on a cotton pad will gently wipe away any make-up without the sting or burn that some chemicals can leave.

11.
Deodorant

Underarms need love too. Give them a break from the chemical clog-up and douse them with some non-toxic treatment for a tropical scent that takes the edge off body odor.

12.
Lip balm/gloss

Whether you want to help heal wind-chaffed or weathered lips or add a dash of glow, coconut oil works wonders.

13.
Bath oil

Add a few tablespoons to your bath with your favorite fragrance and soak it all in. Your skin will feel silky soft without any chemical residue. Truly nature's answer to a spa in a bottle.

14.
Natural hair conditioner & "gel"

Got frizzy, fly-away hair? A drop or two of oil will help soften and control your locks while adding sheen and shine. Massage lightly into the ends, or more towards the root for a deeper conditioning treatment.

For a super deep treatment, wrap in a towel or head your head out into the sunshine for a hot oil treatment that will leave your hair silky soft and healthy looking.

15.
Dandruff control

Massage into scalp and let sit for at least a half an hour. Comb out, rinse, shampoo....then follow with a deep conditioning treatment as mentioned in #14.   Medium chain trigylcerides penetrate the hair shaft, protecting from protein loss.

16.
Shaving

Good-bye razor burn, hello healing coconut oil. Wherever you need a little hair removal, coconut oil will nourish your skin while your shave, penetrating deep into the pore and protect you from any potential ingrown hairs with its antibacterial properties.

Sensual: Nutty love

There are plenty of products out there aimed to "help you out" when the mood strikes. Unfortunately, the unpronounceable list of ingredients alone is enough to make you have an instant headache.

This edible oil is chemical-free, energy-inducing & slippery-smooth with no harmful side-effects on your most private of places. Need we say more?

17.
Massage oil

Non-greasy, non-sticky, smooth and edible. The scent alone will make you feel like you're on a romantic tropical getaway!

18.
Sensual lubricant

Coh!-Coh!-nut oil puts a little more slip in your hitch when you need it.

(Though take fair warning: some research confirms that coconut oil can weaken a latex condom!)

19.
Perfume

Sensitive sniffers with allergies to standard perfumes will appreciate coconut oil's natural scent, boosted by a bevy of other aromatic aromatherapy options. Scents stimulate the limbic system, which in turn, can make certain other systems limber.

Use any of the following essential oils said to increase libido with coconut oil as your base. Black Pepper, Cedarwood, Clary Sage, Clove, Jasmine, Neroli, Patchouli, Pine, Rose, Sandalwood, Vetivert, and Ylang Ylang.

20.
Libido booster

This one might seem like a stretch (pun intended), but trust it...coconut oil's capacity to rev your proverbial engines are indeed a go.

How? Well, low libido can be attributed to a hormonal/ neurotransmitter deficiency, and coconut oil's saturated fats are a precursor for many hormones. Take two tablespoons daily for three weeks and wait for the speedometer to rise.

Pregnancy & nursing: For the mamma in the making

Mothers-to-be can rest easy knowing they are using an all-natural product to assist them in maintaining cravings, keep their skin supple & balance their metabolism. And whatever benefits mamma benefits baby, too.

21.
Immunity booster

Because their bodies are on overdrive, working hard to create that new one within, mothers-to-be tend to be at risk from a host of threatening infections. Coconut oil's lauric acid content has antibacterial, antiviral and antifungal properties, which can boost her immunity and protect her wellness.

22.
Weight balancer

Though weight isn't the first thing a pregnant woman should be concerning herself with, most mamma's in-the-making are a bit worried about gaining too much of it. Eating a sensible diet with coconut oil added in will assist with weight control by promoting the body's ability to burn unwanted fat. Just remember that weight gain is healthy and necessary, for both you and your babe.

23.
Stretch mark reducer & prevention

No pun intended here, but some may think this a terrible stretch. It is said that stretch marks are genetic, and some will get them no matter what they do.

However, it can't hurt to slather it on as your belly begins to stretch, helping to tone the elasticity of your skin (as will upping your doses of vitamin C and E).

Some women claim their lack of stretch marks comes from none other than their daily dose of coconut oil. It is also great for easing the itch that comes with that burgeoning belly and keeping skin there oh-so-soft.

24.
Pre-natal perineum preparation

Now here's a place that will benefit from a little stretching when the big day finally arrives. Your baby's birthday will mark the moment when the perineum will stretch far beyond its typical limits, and hopefully without tearing or the need for surgical cutting (episiotomy).

If you massage your perineum for 5 to 10 minutes a day beginning five or six weeks before your due date, the big stretch will go all that much better.

Add a few drops of lavender oil (to help you relax) to 3 ounces of coconut oil and keep bed-side as a gentle reminder to massage your tender tulip. Better yet, get your honey to do it for you.

25.
Post natal perineum healing and repair

When push comes to shove, you can't always prepare for what's to come. If you do indeed need stitches, postpartum baths and sitz baths speed up healing, and a few drops of coconut oil added to the bath — with its antimicrobial, antifungal and antiviral properties — will prevent infection. It will also help soothe inflammation and any itch from stitches.

Essential oils like lavender, geranium, or cypress will also help tighten severed or stretched tissue and stop bleeding, as well as give a pleasant scent to help you relax and feel rested, which every new mamma needs.

26.
Promotes healthy lactation

Coconut oil is made up of almost 50% lauric acid, the same substance found in mother's milk. It's no secret that mother's milk offers newborns the best protection against viruses, bacteria and protozoa, and most health practitioners encourage new mothers to breastfeed their babies for at least the first year of their life.

So it makes perfect sense that consuming coconut oil, rich in lauric acid, will increase the amount available in her breast milk (some studies say up to three times the original level!)

Other studies indicate that pregnant women, who store fat to assure successful lactation, will also store the lauric acids from her diet, thereby increasing it when she nurses.

Coconut oil also increases its antimicrobial and immune boosting benefits while promoting brain, bone and nerve development in the newborn.

In addition, coconut oil helps soothe and heal tender, cracked nipples without concern of the new baby ingesting any strange chemicals. Gentle massages with a bit of geranium and coconut oil also help soothe sore, lactating breasts.

27.

Ward off gestational diabetes

Some pregnant women experience an elevation of carbohydrate and sugar cravings. Coconut oil helps balance out blood sugar levels, thereby decreasing cravings for foods that aren't good for you or the baby growing inside of you.

28.
Prevents constipation

Pregnant women are known to suffer from constipation, and coconut oil offers a mild laxative-like effect. A little bit of oil taken daily regulates digestion, keeping things moving smoothly.

29.
Soothes hemorrhoids

So much for the pretty glow of pregnancy. If you've not yet invested in the daily intake of coconut oil, your intestines may well be a wadded-up mess and you just can't go. The result is strain and push long before baby comes. Dab a little coconut oil along the inflamed area for immediate relief.

30.
Protects against urinary tract infections

A common ailment during pregnancy, daily intake of coconut oil cleanses the kidneys naturally and gently, preventing the need for antibiotics, which can be dangerous to the newly forming sweet-pea inside you.

31.
Soothes yeast infections

Eases the itch and burn accompanied by yeast infections, common among pregnant women. Apply topically to the inflamed area. Wait. Breathe a big sigh of relief.

Babies: Keeping them pure

While we adults might rationalize the chemicals we ingest, spray or slather on our bodies, a baby's immune system is extra-sensitive. It's up to us to make choices that support their health & wellness.

Coconut oil is all-natural without any harmful side effects. And one easy ingredient added to coconut oil will make all the difference in your little one's world: love!

32.
Diaper rash

Slather a little on and watch the red bumps and inflamed areas disappear in no time at all.

33.
Skin molting

Helps slough off dry, cracked and peeling skin gently and naturally while moisturizing the new skin underneath.

34.
Cradle cap

Moisturize baby's dry and flaking scalp knowing everything that seeps in is positively good for them. Plus, most babies love a gentle head rub!

35.
Heals

Whenever there is an "owie" in our house, our little ones call out for "coco."

Coconut oil can help heal tiny cuts caused by their little fingernails, scraped knees and chaffed areas around the nose during a bout with a cold. We've also used it to help speed healing with insect bites and stings.

36.
Hair tangles & taming

The extra fine baby fuzz at the back of baby's head can get ratty and tattered, making it difficult to comb through. Regularly rub a little coconut oil into the ends and watch the tangles disappear.

For toddlers sporting the wild-child look, add a smidge to their locks to easily tame into place (yes, we wish it worked on the child, too, especially when they are two).

37.
Baby food booster

Did you know medium chain triglycerides or coconut oil are almost always added to commercial baby formulas? Containing almost 50% lauric acid, it's the next best thing to mother's milk.

Add a little to formula and homemade baby food purees or drizzle it on finger foods and watch your little one thrive. With its immune-boosting properties and protection from infections and nutritional diseases, it's a taste they love that loves them back.

38.
Non-toxic massage oil

Whether helping quell colic or simply assisting them in the shift towards nighttime sleep, a baby massaged with coconut oil will help bring peace and quiet for all involved.

Good medicine: No drugstore necessary

Some tout coconut oil as a miracle medicine with a thousand therapeutic uses. There is, as you've previously read, some clear science behind it.

The chemistry of our skin and digestive enzymes help convert coconut oil's medium chain triglycerides into medium chain fatty acid antimicrobials that ward off and destroy potentially damaging fungi, bacteria and viruses.

And that's just the tip of the scientific iceberg.

Look in your medicine cabinet and you're likely to find a slew of products aimed to treat various ailments. If you are leery of smearing topical ointments loaded with ingredients you aren't sure about, why not add coconut oil to your first aid repertoire?

Here are just a few uses for common aches that ail most of us at one time or another.

(For more information on the many other medicinal uses, look to Dr. Bruce Fife, who goes into great detail in his books and website and points towards coconut oil's healing potential for everything from kidney stones to chronic fatigue, with scientific studies and references to support it. www.coconutresearch.org).

39.
Helps heal the skin

Rashes, blisters, cuts, burns, abrasions, cracks- slather on some coconut oil and the healing will speed and soothe all at the same time. The vitamin E found in coconut oil is 40-60 times more powerful than most typical over-the-counter cosmetics and balms, lending to the ease and speed of skin recovery.

40.

Takes the itch out of insect bites

With its anti-inflammatory properties, find relief within minutes of applying coconut oil to most bites or stings. Want to protect yourself from the nasty buggers in the first place? Try a 5:1 Coconut oil to peppermint or lemongrass oil for a homemade insect repellent. Smells a lot better than Deet, don't you think?

41.

Quells the common cold

...while soothing chapped noses & lips. Antimicrobial properties will help the body heal both inside and out.

42.

Soothes and tames a sunburn

Should your tender skin be troubled by a sunburn, slather on some coconut oil for instant relief.

Better yet, protect your skin from the get-go and use coconut oil as you would a sunscreen. Not only does it serve as UV protection, it strengthens the skin and the tissues beneath it.

Detox, energy boost & weight loss: Yes you can!

Coupled with a sensible, well-balanced, whole foods diet filled with plenty of fresh vegetables, fruits and grains, studies show that incorporating coconut oil into your diet can actually help you lose weight.

Try eliminating or lessening most other mainstream oils, cut out sugars, refined flours, processed foods, caffeine, alcohol, and food additives and watch what (and how much) you are eating and see the difference take shape in your shape in no time at all.

A tablespoon two to three times a day can make all the difference in feeling and looking your best.

43.
Stimulates metabolism

The small medium chain triglyceride molecules make the oil light and thereby lighten the load to your digestive system, allowing enzymes to digest medium chain fatty acids easily. The result? A higher metabolic rate, and a body that burns fat naturally.

44.
Reduces hunger

The fats in coconut oil help your belly feel full sooner so you don't overeat. Couple that with the yogic notion of eating only two palm-fulls of food (preferably one palm of grain, the other of vegetables) and add the "five minute rule" (stop eating for five minutes after eating a reasonable portion of food) to each meal and you'll likely see that you truly ARE full, after all.

45.
Balances blood sugar

Coconut oil improves digestion and absorption of fat-soluble vitamins, minerals (especially calcium and magnesium), and amino acids. It improves the body's use of blood glucose and improves insulin secretion and absorption.

46.
Improves digestive functions

Because it is easily absorbed by your body, coconut oil takes some of the strain off of your digestive system and aids in the absorption of essential vitamins and minerals. It also expels wastes & toxins by nourishing cells.

47.

Detox with oil pulling

The health of our mouth is critical in keeping up with the wellness in our overall health, because, believe it or not, most diseases begin there!

Derived from Ayurvedic traditions, oil pulling cleanses the mouth by removing the toxins from the mouth, teeth and tongue.

Take one tablespoon of coconut oil then gently pull and swish the oil over the teeth and gums for fifteen to twenty minutes.

This swishing activates the enzymes which in turn draws the toxins out of the blood. Spit out that mouthful of spittle, rinse with warm water and repeat each day, first thing, on an empty stomach.

Another easy way to say yes to your health and hello to a happy mouth.

Pets: TLC for our fluffy friends

Don't forget your four legged friends! Most animals love the taste of coconut oil and benefit from it in most of the ways we do, so adding it to their daily repertoire will keep them happy and healthy in a preventative and proactive way without any negative side affects.

While coconut oil is a great support for your pet's wellness and health, serious medical issues should always be brought to the attention of your pet's vet.

48.

Add it to their food

They'll benefit in all the ways we humans do. Be sure to add only a small amount, as some animals are more finicky to new tastes than others (though one of our cats licks it right off my finger!) and too much too soon could cause loose stools. Consult your veterinarian for recommended dosage amounts, as pet sizes and needs vary, though some recommend working up to 1 tsp. per every ten pounds a day.

49.
Helps with hairballs

The natural lubrication of coconut oil helps our critters cough up what gets stuck. Your pet will also benefit from the shine while also helping with any dry skin issues. A half a teaspoon every few days usually does the trick with our super finicky cat, though I'm certain our other cat would drink the whole jar if we'd let her.

50.
Cures cuts & minor infections

Dab a little bit of oil on small cuts and monitor any infections. The antiviral and antimicrobial affects help speed the healing.

House, home & otherwise...

So if you're going to take a healthy lifestyle plunge, you might as well add non-toxic cleaning supplies to your daily repertoire. Rid your pantry and garage of those scary cans of chemicals and replace with a large jar of coconut oil for all your grease, grime, rust, corrosion and lubrication needs. A spray bottle of white vinegar, some baking soda, some old dust rags and a scrub brush, a bucket of water and some good ol' fashioned elbow grease are just about all you need to make things sparkle and shine without any chemical residual grime.

51.
Overall lubricant

From bicycle chains to luggage zippers to keyholes to all your hand held garden tools, coconut oil will help keep your things from getting stuck or rusty.

52.
Squeak removal

The squeaky wheel will get the oil. So will the door hinge, that creaky gate, your swivel chair, the kid's swing-set chains, the weathervane. Up, down, all around — if it squeaks, coconut oil's got you covered.

53.
Degreasing agent

Clean up the grease and grime from just about any slick surface. A dab'll do. Just add elbow grease applied with a nice clean cloth.

54.
Sports aid

Keep your gear in check while you play. Protects the leather on your baseball glove, polishes your lucky fishing lure, keeps the rust from your ice skate blades, shines up your bowling ball, lubes up your skateboard trucks, polishes your pool stick, protects your kite line, greases up your bike chain, lubes up your wetsuit zipper, your sailboat sheaves, your roller skates. Surf, sand, sea, land, bowling alley lanes…wherever you play, coconut oil is on your team.

55.
Non-putrifying polisher

Shine those shoes, buff up those boots. Polish your great aunt Bea's wooden violin and make the old oak table glow for that family sit-down meal. Condition that saddle, that belt, those winter gloves — coconut oil won't go rancid, so it's safe to use and smells good, too.

56.
Marine lubricant

To keep your boat ship shape (and the stuff aboard it), turn to coconut oil's many maritime uses. Salt corrosion protection on rubber molding and console panel switches, freely spinning fishing reels, easy, usable on-board hand tools, and teak with a buffed up beauty—this tropical topical will aid you and all that is sea-worthy.

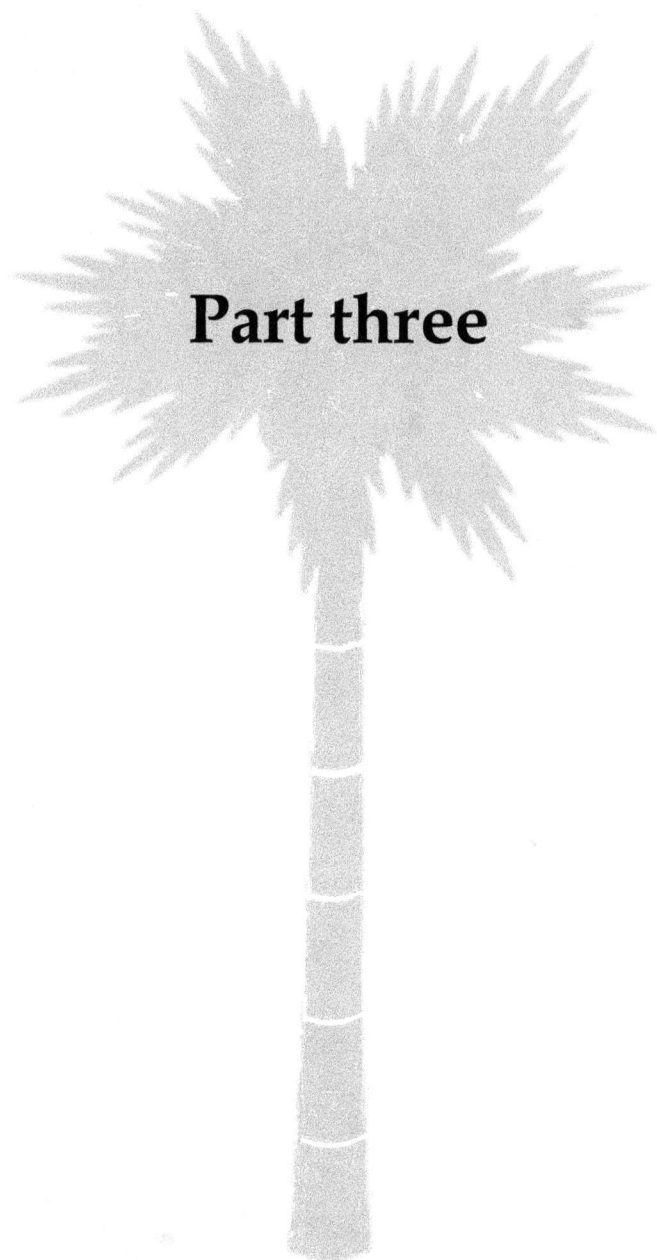

Part three

Powerful prescription & defense against disease

When your state of health is compromised, you do all you can to create better balance within. This book isn't meant to be cavalier towards those that struggle with serious medical issues, nor is it meant to replace any medical counseling, medications or serve as a stand-alone treatment for any serious health conditions you may be suffering from.

What has been offered so far is information, in an easy-to-use fashion, about coconut oil and all that it can do to support you towards health and wellness.

Coconut oil is, after all, a food and not a drug, and when mindfully applied within a balanced lifestyle — provides a harmless and inexpensive way to propagate wellness within our own bodies. Only you (and your health care provider) know what's best for you — we encourage you to explore the uses and decide what resonates.

That said, do know that research continues to show how this natural remedy aids in some very serious diseases and chronic infections WITHOUT ANY HARMFUL SIDE EFFECTS. Dr. Bruce Fife and several others have done scores of research and collected testimonials to show that

according to research, coconut oil use can assist with the following:

Diabetes.

Heart disease.

Thyroid function.

Fungal infections.

Stomach ulcers & hyperacidity.

Urinary tract infections.

Kidney stones.

Pneumonia.

Gonnorhoea (STD's).

Intestinal worms.

Tumors.

Heartburn, acid reflux & indigestion.

Chronic fatigue syndrome.

Antiviral activity for influenza, herpes, measles, hepatitis C, SARS, HIV & many other viruses.

Kidney, gallbladder & liver disease.

Chronic inflammation.

Eczema & psoriasis.

Ringworm, scabies, lice.

Warts and moles.

Gingivitis.

Gum disease.
Scurvy.

Toothaches, periodontal disease & tooth decay.

Migraines.

Skin and nail fungus.

Aging spots.

Arthritis.

Candida.

And much, much more.

Since I am neither scientist nor doctor, and can only go on my own personal experience of dealing with Candida and none of the other problems mentioned above, I cannot authentically write about the miraculous curing effects of coconut oil in each instance. There are, however, more than hundreds of such testimonials written in books listed in the reference section of this book, and countless scientific studies currently being done to further investigate the facts.

If you are someone who in fact suffers from some of the above troublesome infections or serious diseases, perhaps the references will be of some assistance to you along your road to recovery.

Hope coupled with clear and helpful information can go a very long way.

Last but not least... Give it time

If you are simply trying coconut oil for it's pleasurable effects and amazing basic daily uses, have at it! But if you are exploring coconut oil for more dire needs, consult your doctor, and by all means, be easy on yourself. Studies show it at least takes three weeks for any new pattern to become habituated in the mind and body, so go slow and steady, and do what's necessary to support yourself on that path.

Coconut oil is NOT a cure-all, but it IS an amazing cure for many ailments, and when coupled with proper diet, lifestyle, attitude and exercise, it can prove to be extremely effective for most who try it.

Now here's the tough news you may or may not already know: Sometimes people feel worse before they feel better when they start to "cleanse." Detoxification is tricky like that.

Your body needs time to process and eliminate all the toxins it might be holding — and might have been holding for quite some time. Your kidneys will be hard at work for you as will your skin and liver.

Drink lots of water, rest when necessary, eat whole, organic foods and partake in some form of daily physical activity to help keep the blood pumping, your cells oxygenated and your breath smooth and fluid.

You might even choose to explore other alternative options to assist you, such as massage therapy, acupuncture, energy healing, chiropractic treatments, colonics, yoga, and meditation— all modalities that can lend a hand in helping you balance your energy.

Or you might choose to hire a personal trainer, nutritional counselor or wellness coach to help you feel empowered and encouraged while you work towards wellness.

The true key to health is not just only in what certain foods you do or do not eat or what exercise you do and how much you do it, but in learning how to balance your energy to its most beneficial potential in your present time situation. What worked for you yesterday might not feel so great today and vice versa. Tune IN and see what's what.

Your choices add up over a lifetime—when you come to truly understand that these choices are yours and yours alone to make, you will inevitably become more conscious and sensitive of their negative and positive impacts.

Some of us will be more propelled than others to go full tilt and lean deeply into a pure and clean diet and lifestyle. Others, myself included, will aim for that but fall more into a happy medium within our mainstream society, relishing in the occasional decadent pastry and con leche while still maintaining a standard set of health "rules of the road." Happiness and health do not come in a one size fits all equation, and it's up to you to figure out what the balance will be.

This book isn't written to be

condemning of any of the choices you make, but simply to offer you easy options in maximizing your fullest potential if it is calling out to you.

Here's to you and all that you choose in this precious life. May it support you along your way.

Resources & references

Most of the research I've done during the last five years has been gathered from a combination of books, the web and simple personal use.

Interestingly, I've found less than ten books on coconut oil. The amount of information on the web, however, has multiplied thousand-fold in the last five years! The many benefits of this oil are starting to be truly comprehended — with studies being done and information made available from them proof that the coconut oil train has left the proverbial station.

I have not listed each individual study or abstract I've read in the last five years, but the following references are where most are located and are a great place to begin for more information.

Books

Coconut Oil: For Health and Beauty by Cynthia Holzapfel, Laura Holzapfel

Coconut Oil: Rev Up Your System-Change Your Oil! by Barbara Wexler

Coconut Oil: Discover the Key to Vibrant Health by Siegfried Gursche

The Coconut Oil Miracle by Bruce Fife

Virgin Cocount Oil: Nature's Miracle Medicine by Bruce Fife

Virgin Coconut Oil: How It Has Changed People's Lives, and How It Can Change Yours! by Brian Shilhavy, Marianita Jader Shilhavy,

Websites

coconutresearchcenter.org
Dr. Fife explores and discusses much- if not most- of the scientific studies & abstracts on coconut oil here on this prolific site.

coconutoil.com
Another fantastic site showcasing scientific studies, abstracts, reports & testimonials. They consider themselves the leading website on the most current research on the health benefits of coconut oil.

loc.gov./rr/scitech/mysteries/coconut

foodallergy.org

earthclinic.com

naturalnews.com

Products

There are many fantastic products out there and part of the enjoyment and empowerment of healing comes from checking it out for yourself. Most health food stores will carry at least a brand or two of virgin oils, and even some major grocery stores now stock a brand on their shelves, as well. Just be sure they are virgin, unbleached, non-hydrogenated and unrefined. It helps globally if they are fair trade and fair wage, too.

That said, here are a couple of companies I've found to offer high quality products with integrity in both production and distribution. I have no financial affiliations with either.

www.nutiva.com
www.vivapura.com

About the Author

Cricket Desmarais is a writer and yoga instructor living with her family in Key West, Florida.

She is dedicated to living—and helping others live— a more luminous and joyful life, as simply and sanely as possible.

For more information on Cricket and her other books and creative projects, visit: **www.cricketdesmarais.com** & **www.ilovecoconutoil.com.**